The Power of Pause

Unleashing the Benefits of Intermittent Fasting

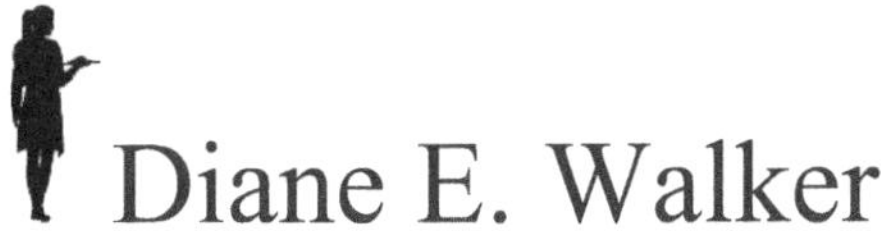

Diane E. Walker

TABLE OF CONTENTS

INTRODUCTION...7

CHAPTER ONE...11

Intermittent Fasting 11

Some Of the Advantages of Intermittent Fasting

....13

The History of Intermittent Fasting 15

How Intermittent Fasting Works.....................21

Is It Possible That Intermittent Fasting Is the Best

Option for You? 24

CHAPTER TWO 29

The Science of Intermittent Fasting.................29

The Physiological Underpinnings of Starvation

and Fullness..32

Insulin's Importance in the Context of

Intermittent Fasting 34

The Advantages of Undergoing Autophagy 39

Some Possible Advantages of the Process of Autophagy 43

The Research That Supports Weight Loss and a Healthy Metabolism 45

The Effects of Periodic Fasting on the Aging Process and the Length of One's Life 50

The Effects of Periodic Fasting on the Health of the Brain and Its Capacity for Cognitive Function 55

CHAPTER THREE **61**

Different Approaches to Intermittent Fasting ..61

Time-Restricted Feeding 63

Alternate-day fasting (ADF) 66

5:2 Abstinence and Fasting 71

Spontaneous Meal Skipping 74

Combining Fasting with Other Diets to Achieve Your Health Goals....................................79

CHAPTER FOUR...................................**84**

Implementing Intermittent Fasting into Your Lifestyle...84

How to Get Started with the Health Benefits of Intermittent Fasting..............................84

How to Get Ready for Fasting Periods That Are Spaced Apart.......................................88

Managing Hunger and Cravings......................93

What to Consume for Food and Drink Throughout the Fasting Period........................98

How to Break the Fast Without Risking Your Health...103

Overcoming Obstacles That Are Often Encountered..105

CHAPTER FIVE...................................**112**

The Future of Intermittent Fasting 112

The Most Recent Studies and Fast-Developing Trends 114

The Possible Therapeutic Benefits of Periodic Fasting for several Different Health Conditions 119

The Importance of Periodic Fasting in the Field of Preventative Medicine 121

CONCLUSION 124

What Steps Should Be Taken Next: Websites that provide resources for more information and support 127

INTRODUCTION

In recent years, intermittent fasting has been an increasingly well-known method for achieving weight reduction and bettering one's overall health. It consists of alternating times of eating with periods of fasting, and there are many various ways to incorporate it into your lifestyle to get the desired effects. Yet beyond merely being a fad diet, research has proven that intermittent fasting provides several health and wellness advantages that are beneficial to the individual as a whole.

In this book, we will investigate the science that lies behind intermittent fasting as well as its effects on both the body and the mind. We will discuss the several ways that intermittent fasting may be done, how you can incorporate it into your lifestyle, and what you can anticipate as you embark on this path. As individuals attempt intermittent fasting for the first time, they often have questions, worries, and difficulties that we will discuss.

This book will offer you all of the knowledge you want to get started with intermittent fasting, regardless of whether you are interested in it to prevent illness, lose weight, or just feeling better and living longer. Now that we have established that, let's go further and investigate the power of pausing, also known as the power of intermittent fasting.

In the next chapters, we will investigate the science underpinning intermittent fasting and how it operates in more depth. We are going to investigate the physiological processes that take place during fasting, such as autophagy and insulin control, as well as how these processes contribute to the health advantages of intermittent fasting.

In addition, we are going to take a more in-depth look at the various methods of intermittent fasting, such as time-restricted eating, alternate-day fasting, 5:2 fasting, and modified fasting. We'll go through the benefits and drawbacks of each strategy, as well as how to evaluate them and decide which one could work best for you.

If you're accustomed to eating at regular intervals throughout the day, incorporating intermittent fasting into your lifestyle might be a challenge. This is particularly true if you're trying to lose weight. Because of this, we are going to provide you with some helpful advice and techniques that will make the practice of intermittent fasting simpler and more manageable. We will discuss how to deal with feelings of hunger and cravings, what kinds of foods and beverages are acceptable throughout the fasting time, and how to break the fast healthily.

In the last part of this series, we will talk about the future of intermittent fasting and the possible health advantages that it may have for a variety of illnesses. In addition to that, we will provide you with sites where you can get further knowledge and assistance so that you may continue your journey of intermittent fasting with complete assurance.

This book will equip you with the information and resources you need to make the most of this effective method for optimizing your health, regardless of whether you are just starting with intermittent fasting or are an experienced practitioner of the technique. Now that we understand the importance of pausing to improve our health, let's get started on the path.

CHAPTER ONE

Intermittent Fasting

Alternating intervals of eating with periods in which one does not consume any food is the basis of the diet strategy known as "intermittent fasting." The goal of this strategy is to accomplish several health advantages, including weight reduction, increased insulin sensitivity, and lower inflammation, by limiting calorie consumption during certain periods of the day or week.

There are a few distinct methods for carrying out intermittent fasting, but they all require either time-restricted food or fasting for longer periods at regular intervals. Time-restricted feeding is reducing the amount of time you spend eating each day to a certain number of hours, such as eight hours, and then going without food for the other 16 hours of the day. On the other hand, periodic fasting is abstaining from food and drink for extended periods, often twenty-four or more hours, regularly. The practice of intermittent fasting may be carried out in a variety of various ways; nevertheless, it is essential to choose a method that is suitable for both your unique requirements and your way of life. Some individuals find that beginning with shorter fasting times is simpler, while others may feel that longer fasting intervals are more beneficial.

In general, intermittent fasting is not a diet in the conventional sense of the word; rather, it refers to a pattern of eating that includes alternating times of eating with periods of not eating. It has the potential to be a useful instrument for enhancing your health and well-being, provided you go about it properly and get some assistance.

In many different cultures and faiths, including Islam, Judaism, Christianity, and Buddhism, the practice of fasting for periods that are not consecutive has been observed for many centuries. Because of the expanding amount of data that substantiates its advantages, it has seen a meteoric rise in popularity in recent years as a method for achieving both weight reduction and overall health improvement.

Some Of the Advantages of Intermittent Fasting

Weight Reduction: Weight reduction is a potential benefit of intermittent fasting, which works by limiting the amount of time each day that a person is allowed to consume food. This, in turn, helps decrease overall calorie consumption.

Increased Insulin Sensitivity: Intermittent fasting has been shown to help increase insulin sensitivity, which in turn may result in lower blood sugar levels and a decreased chance of developing type 2 diabetes.

Decreased inflammation Research: Decreased inflammation Research has indicated that intermittent fasting may lower levels of inflammation in the body, which is important since inflammation is a risk factor for a wide variety of chronic illnesses.

Increased Autophagy: Intermittent fasting has been shown to boost autophagy, which is a process that occurs inside cells that helps eliminate damaged cells and promotes cellular rejuvenation.

Increased Brain Function: Research has revealed that intermittent fasting may increase brain function and protect against neurodegenerative disorders. While there are numerous potential advantages to intermittent fasting, it is crucial to keep in mind that it may not be appropriate for everyone. Before beginning the practice of intermittent fasting, women who are pregnant or nursing, persons who have a history of eating disorders, and those who have specific medical problems should discuss the practice with their primary care physician.

The History of Intermittent Fasting

The idea of fasting on an intermittent basis is not a new one and has been around for thousands of years in a variety of different ways. A variety of societies and faiths all over the world have embraced the practice of fasting in some shape or another as part of their customs and rituals.

One of the oldest kinds of fasting that has been recorded goes back to ancient Greece. Throughout that period, people in Greece thought that fasting might heal a variety of maladies. Hippocrates, who is widely regarded as the "father" of modern medicine, suggested that those who were sick should abstain from food as a kind of therapy.

Moreover, fasting has played a significant role in the practice of many religious traditions. One of the Five Pillars of Islam is abstaining from food and drink throughout the month of Ramadan. This obligation applies to all healthy people over the age of 18. In the Christian religion, abstaining from food and drink for a period called Lent, which lasts for forty days before Easter, is common practice. On many days throughout the year, including Yom Kippur, also known as the Day of Atonement, followers of Judaism observe the practice of fasting. Fasting on and off at regular intervals is one method that has been utilized to boost athletic performance. Before taking part in games, athletes in ancient Greece would fast in order to strengthen their physical capabilities. Bodybuilders and other athletes have turned to intermittent fasting in recent years as a means of increasing their muscle mass while simultaneously decreasing their overall body fat percentage.

The use of intermittent fasting as a method for reducing excess body fat and improving overall health has seen a meteoric rise in popularity in the contemporary period. The expanding corpus of research on intermittent fasting has served to verify the advantages of this practice and has contributed to the practice becoming more prevalent in modern society.

Nowadays, there are a variety of techniques for intermittent fasting, and the topic continues to be one that is the focus of study and attention among both medical professionals and laypeople who are interested in improving their health.

In recent years, research on intermittent fasting has seen substantial expansion, and there is now a substantial body of scientific data supporting the claims that it is beneficial to both one's health and well-being.

Dr. Clive McKay of Cornell University is credited with carrying out one of the early investigations on intermittent fasting, which took place in the 1940s. He discovered that rats who were given food every other day lived longer and were in better health than rats that were free to eat whatever they wanted whenever they wanted (whenever they wanted). Since then, a large number of further research have been conducted to investigate the effects of intermittent fasting on both human and animal subjects.

In recent years, a number of large-scale human investigations have been conducted, and the results of this research have offered compelling evidence of the advantages of intermittent fasting. Alternate-day fasting was shown to lead to considerable weight reduction and better indices of cardiovascular health, such as blood pressure and cholesterol levels, according to research that was published in the New England Journal of Medicine. An additional study that was published in the journal Cell Metabolism discovered that time-restricted feeding, which is an approach to intermittent fasting that involves limiting eating to a specific time window each day, improved insulin sensitivity and reduced blood pressure in overweight adults who had metabolic syndrome.

Fasting on an as-needed basis has also been proven to have anti-aging benefits, with research conducted on animals indicating that it may be able to lengthen lifespan and enhance health outcomes associated with aging.

Researchers believe that improvements in metabolic function, cellular repair processes, and hormonal regulation may be related to the benefits of intermittent fasting. While the exact mechanisms behind the benefits of intermittent fasting are not yet fully understood, researchers believe that they may be related.

In general, the expanding corpus of research on intermittent fasting shows that it may be a useful technique for enhancing both one's health and overall well-being. Nonetheless, similar to making any other changes to one's diet or way of life, it is essential to approach intermittent fasting with prudence and to confer with a healthcare professional before beginning the practice.

It is essential to keep in mind that intermittent fasting is not a silver bullet and is not intended to serve as a replacement for a balanced diet or way of life. Yet, when used in combination with other healthy behaviors, it has the potential to become a potent instrument for enhancing both one's health and well-being. Any modification to one's diet or way of life should, as a matter of course, be approached with prudence, and one should confer with a healthcare professional before getting started.

How Intermittent Fasting Works

In order for intermittent fasting to be effective, there must be a caloric deficit in the body. This shortfall, in turn, may result in weight reduction and an improvement in metabolic health. The practice of intermittent fasting may be carried out in a number of distinct ways; however, the one that is practiced most often involves limiting food consumption to certain windows of time or days of the week.

Time-restricted feeding, also known as time-restricted eating, is a technique of intermittent fasting that entails restricting the amount of time each day during which one consumes food to a certain window. For instance, a person may choose to limit their eating to the period of time between noon and eight o'clock in the evening, and then abstain from food for the other 16 hours of the day. Since it consists of a fasting phase of 16 hours followed by an eating window of 8 hours, this strategy is sometimes referred to as the 16:8 technique.

Alternate-day fasting is a kind of intermittent fasting that includes eating normally on one day and then reducing the amount of food consumed to a very low level (often about 500 calories) on the following day. This type of fasting is performed in cycles. This strategy could be more difficult, but it might result in more significant weight reduction and increased metabolic advantages.

When a person goes without food for an extended length of time, their bodies switch from utilizing glucose (sugar) as a source of energy to utilizing stored fat instead. When glucose is not readily accessible, the body will burn fat reserves for energy instead of using glucose, which might result in weight loss. It has also been shown that fasting may enhance insulin sensitivity and decrease inflammation, both of which can lead to improved metabolic health and a lower chance of developing chronic illnesses such as diabetes and cardiovascular disease.

Alterations in hormone levels are another potential effect of intermittent fasting. These changes may include an increase in the synthesis of human growth hormone (HGH) and a reduction in insulin levels. Although insulin is responsible for the storage of fat in the body, human growth hormone (HGH) plays a crucial role in the maintenance of muscle mass and the promotion of fat burning. Intermittent fasting may help the body burn fat more effectively by lowering insulin levels. This occurs as a result of decreased insulin production.

Is It Possible That Intermittent Fasting Is the Best Option for You?

It is not easy to provide a response to such a question. In general, it is essential to think about why you want to experiment with intermittent fasting and what you want to get out of the experience. Do you intend to continue doing this for the rest of your life?

There are a lot of individuals who attempt to lose weight by fasting, but if it's not something you can do permanently – or if the strategy isn't sustainable - it's possible that you will gain all of the weight back. A possible benefit of intermittent fasting for weight reduction is that it may encourage you to consume fewer calories on a daily basis. This is particularly true if you eat sensibly during periods when you are not fasting and pick meals that are nutritionally sound.

Take a minute to reflect on the way in which you typically eat. If you find that you snack a lot late at night and want to eat less, intermittent fasting may help you set a limit for yourself and force you to eat fewer meals overall. If you find that you finish your final meal of the day late in the evening, consider eating earlier in the day to give your body the opportunity to begin the fasting process sooner.

In general, the precise processes that underlie the advantages of intermittent fasting are not yet completely known; nonetheless, research indicates that it may be a useful strategy for enhancing health and well-being. It is vital to approach intermittent fasting with prudence and to check with a healthcare physician before beginning the practice, just as it is necessary to approach any change in diet or lifestyle.

Intermittent fasting may help decrease inflammation in the body, which may play a role in the development of chronic illnesses such as heart disease, cancer, and arthritis. In addition to the advantages that were described previously, intermittent fasting may also help reduce inflammation in the body. Intermittent fasting may help guard against chronic illnesses and boost general health and well-being by lowering the levels of inflammation in the body.

By boosting insulin sensitivity, intermittent fasting may also help minimize the chance of developing type 2 diabetes, which is another benefit of this eating pattern. Insulin is a hormone that controls how much sugar is in the blood in the human body. When insulin sensitivity is poor, the body has a harder time reacting to insulin, which may lead to high blood sugar levels and an increased risk of type 2 diabetes. When insulin sensitivity is low, the chance of developing type 2 diabetes also increases. Intermittent fasting may help lower the likelihood of developing diabetes by increasing insulin sensitivity, which is one of the disease's risk factors. One other mechanism by which intermittent fasting may be effective is via the promotion of autophagy, which is the process by which the body degrades and recycles damaged or aged cells. It has been shown that autophagy provides anti-aging effects as well as anti-cancer benefits, and it may also assist enhance general health and lifespan.

It is essential to keep in mind that despite the fact that intermittent fasting has shown promise as a method for enhancing one's health and well-being, it is not a panacea. It is essential to combine intermittent fasting with other healthy behaviors, such as regular exercise and a diet that is balanced and rich in nutrients, in order to get the full advantages of this practice. In addition, it is essential that you pay attention to your body and make any necessary adjustments to your fasting schedule in order to guarantee that you are able to satisfy your nutritional requirements and keep your weight in a healthy range.

CHAPTER TWO

The Science of Intermittent Fasting

Researchers are currently studying the science underlying intermittent fasting; nevertheless, they have uncovered many pathways that may explain how intermittent fasting works to enhance health and promote weight reduction.

Alterations in the hormonal equilibrium of the body are one of the key effects that may be brought about by practicing intermittent fasting. When we eat, our bodies secrete insulin, which assists in moving glucose from circulation into the cells where it may be used as a source of energy. Additionally, insulin assists the body in converting excess glucose into fat stores. When we don't eat for an extended period of time, our insulin levels decrease, and our bodies start using the fat they have stored as fuel instead of glucose. This may result in a reduction in body fat and an improvement in metabolic health.

It is possible that the practice of intermittent fasting works by elevating levels of human growth hormone (HGH), a hormone that contributes to the reduction of body fat and the development of new muscle. According to a number of studies, intermittent fasting may lead to a significant rise in human growth hormone (HGH) levels, which in turn can enhance both body composition and athletic performance.

Additionally, there is some evidence that intermittent fasting might help decrease inflammation in the body, which is a factor that has been linked to the development of a wide variety of chronic illnesses. Intermittent fasting may help protect against illnesses such as heart disease, cancer, and arthritis by lowering overall levels of inflammation in the body.

In addition, there is some evidence that intermittent fasting might aid boost the body's cellular repair mechanisms, namely a process known as autophagy. Autophagy is the process through which the body eliminates damaged cells and recycles waste from cellular metabolism. It has been shown to offer anti-aging advantages as well as anti-cancer properties, and it may also assist boost general health and lifespan.

Even though the science underpinning intermittent fasting is still being developed, there is growing evidence that the practice may be an effective method for enhancing health and facilitating weight reduction. However, it is essential to keep in mind that intermittent fasting may not be suitable for everyone and that further study is required to get a comprehensive understanding of both the possible advantages and hazards associated with it. Before making any major changes to your diet or lifestyle, it is important to discuss your plans with a qualified medical professional.

The Physiological Underpinnings of Starvation and Fullness

Both hunger and fullness are intricate physiological processes that are controlled in the body by a variety of hormones and neurotransmitters.

The hormone known as ghrelin, which is secreted by the stomach, is an important player in the process of controlling hunger. When the stomach is empty, levels of the hormone ghrelin increase, which sends a message to the brain that it is time to eat. The levels of the hormone leptin increase after we eat, which sends a message to the brain that we are no longer hungry and should stop eating. Insulin, which is secreted in reaction to eating, has a function in the regulation of hunger and fullness by contributing to the regulation of blood sugar levels and controlling appetite. Insulin is released in response to eating.

Other variables, in addition to these hormonal signals, may have an effect on one's level of hunger or satiety. For instance, the sight, smell, and taste of food may induce hunger, even though the body does not need to require more calories. This is because food stimulates the senses of sight, smell, and taste. On the other hand, things like stress, worry, and sadness may decrease appetite and contribute to sensations of fullness, even if the body is in need of food. This can happen even if the individual hasn't eaten in a while.

Hunger and satiety are processes that, in general, are very personalized and may be impacted by a variety of variables, including heredity, the environment, and the habits that people have in their daily lives. It can be helpful to develop strategies to manage hunger and promote satiety by gaining an understanding of the physiological mechanisms that underlie these processes. Some of these strategies include consuming a diet that is balanced and contains a sufficient amount of protein and fiber, drinking a sufficient amount of water, and avoiding highly processed foods, which can disrupt hormonal balance and lead to overeating.

Insulin's Importance in the Context of Intermittent Fasting

Insulin is a hormone that is essential to the process of controlling the amount of sugar that is present in the blood in the body. During the process of digestion, the carbohydrates in the food we consume are converted into glucose, which is subsequently made available in circulation. In reaction, the pancreas secretes insulin, a hormone that assists in the movement of glucose from circulation into the cells of the body, where it may be used for energy or stored. This process contributes to the maintenance of normal levels of blood sugar and supplies the body with the energy it needs in order to operate normally.

When a person goes without food for an extended amount of time, their insulin levels decrease, and their bodies start using the glucose they have stored as fat for energy. This may result in a reduction in body fat and an improvement in metabolic health. In addition, there is some evidence that intermittent fasting might assist enhance insulin sensitivity, which makes it simpler for the body to react to insulin and maintain stable blood sugar levels.

However, it is essential to keep in mind that insulin plays a multifaceted function in the body; hence, lowering insulin levels alone is not necessarily the solution to improve one's health. In point of fact, a number of studies have shown that having insulin levels that are persistently low may result in insulin resistance as well as other health issues.

Additionally, people who have diabetes or other medical conditions that affect insulin regulation should always consult with a healthcare provider prior to attempting intermittent fasting or making significant changes to their diet or lifestyle. This is because these kinds of changes can have serious consequences for insulin regulation.

When it comes to comprehending the advantages of intermittent fasting, insulin is only one piece of the jigsaw. This is despite the fact that insulin plays a significant part in the regulation of both the metabolism and the levels of blood sugar. Intermittent fasting may help enhance metabolic health and lower the chance of developing chronic illnesses like diabetes and heart disease by increasing insulin sensitivity and encouraging healthy hormonal balance. However, as is the case when making any kind of modification to one's diet or way of life, it is critical to pay attention to how your body reacts, to discuss the matter with a medical professional, and to be flexible enough to make adjustments as required to ensure that your nutritional requirements are met and that you keep a healthy weight.

Insulin is essential for the breakdown and use of fat, in addition to its function in controlling the amount of sugar in the blood. When insulin levels are high, the body is in an anabolic condition, which means that it is storing energy and developing new tissues. This is the opposite of a catabolic state, which occurs when insulin levels are low. People who are working on increasing their muscle mass or their overall body mass might stand to benefit from this. On the other hand, if insulin levels remain raised for an extended period of time, the body may develop a resistance to the effects of the hormone, which may result in weight gain, inflammation, and other health issues.

It has been suggested that intermittent fasting may assist increase insulin sensitivity, so enabling the body to react to insulin in a more efficient manner and lowering the risk of insulin resistance as well as other metabolic problems. Intermittent fasting may assist enhance the body's capacity to metabolize glucose and fat by providing the body with a break from its continual production of insulin. This, in turn, may lead to increased levels of energy, weight reduction, and better overall health.

In addition, there is some evidence that intermittent fasting might assist in the reduction of inflammation in the body, which is yet another important aspect of metabolic health. Inflammation is a normal reaction to an injury or infection; nevertheless, persistent inflammation may lead to a wide variety of health issues, including coronary heart disease, type 2 diabetes, and cancer. Intermittent fasting has been shown in certain studies to help decrease inflammation in the body by controlling the production of inflammatory cytokines and other immune components.

Even though insulin plays a complicated part in intermittent fasting, there is accumulating evidence to show that this kind of fasting may be an effective approach for improving metabolic health and lowering the risk of developing chronic illnesses. However, just as it is essential to talk with a healthcare expert before making any changes to your diet or lifestyle, you should do the same to verify that you are fulfilling your nutritional requirements and keeping a healthy weight after making any changes to your diet or lifestyle.

The Advantages of Undergoing Autophagy

Autophagy is a natural process that occurs in the body that involves the dismantling and recycling of cellular components that have become dysfunctional or damaged. This process helps to maintain healthy cells and ensures that they perform as they should, and it has been connected to a variety of health advantages.

It has been found to promote autophagy in the body, which may assist improve general health and lower the chance of developing chronic illnesses. Intermittent fasting has been demonstrated to increase autophagy in the body.

In addition, there is evidence to indicate that autophagy may possibly play a part in the process of delaying the aging process. Our cells become more damaged and dysfunctional as we get older, which may lead to a wide variety of illnesses and ailments that are associated with aging. Autophagy is a process that assists the body in removing damaged cellular components, which in turn lessens the load of cellular damage and may possibly slow down the aging process.

Some studies have even hypothesized that autophagy might be the key to unlocking the anti-aging advantages of calorie restriction and intermittent fasting. These dietary treatments may help minimize cellular damage and increase cellular function, ultimately leading to better health and lifespan. This is achieved by stimulating autophagy, which in turn is achieved by promoting autophagy. However, despite the fact that autophagy has been associated with a variety of positive impacts on health, it is essential to stress that further study is required in order to completely understand the processes that are responsible for these effects. Additionally, it is crucial to approach any dietary intervention with caution and to check with a healthcare expert before making large changes to either your diet or your lifestyle. This is especially important if you are pregnant or breastfeeding. Even while it has been shown to be safe and helpful for a large number of individuals, intermittent fasting may not be suitable for everyone, especially those who have certain medical issues or dietary requirements.

Autophagy may also be beneficial to the immune system, which is another possible advantage of this process. It has been shown that autophagy plays a significant part in the process of eliminating damaged or diseased cells, and it is of special significance for the upkeep of the health of immune cells.

The study has shown that autophagy may help enhance immune function by boosting the body's capacity to identify and react to external invaders like viruses and bacteria. This research implies that autophagy may assist improve immunological function.

In addition, autophagy has the potential to help minimize the risk of developing autoimmune illnesses by removing damaged immune cells, which are known to contribute to the development of these ailments.

There is some evidence that autophagy plays a part in the process of keeping the brain and nervous system healthy. According to the findings of a few pieces of research, autophagy has the potential to aid in the removal of harmful proteins that may build up in the brain over time and contribute to illnesses such as Alzheimer's disease and Parkinson's disease.

Some Possible Advantages of the Process of Autophagy

Enhanced performance of individual cells: Autophagy is a process that may assist enhance cellular function and lower the risk of cellular damage and malfunction. This is accomplished by degrading and recycling cellular components that have been damaged.

Reduced inflammation: It has been shown that autophagy may reduce inflammation in the body by degrading inflammatory proteins and removing damaged cells.

Improved metabolic health: Increased insulin sensitivity may be reduced, and both glucose and lipid metabolism may be improved as a result of autophagy, according to the findings of some research.

Reduced risk of chronic diseases: Autophagy has been related to a lower risk of chronic illnesses such as cancer, Alzheimer's disease, and Parkinson's disease. This is because autophagy breaks down dead cells and recycles their components.

Overall, although more research is required to fully understand the role that autophagy plays in both health and disease, there is growing evidence to suggest that promoting autophagy through interventions such as intermittent fasting may have important health benefits. This is despite the fact that more research is needed to fully understand the role that autophagy plays. However, before making any changes to your diet or lifestyle, it is vital to talk with a healthcare expert. This is especially important if you have any preexisting medical issues or are already taking medication.

The Research That Supports Weight Loss and a Healthy Metabolism

It has been shown that intermittent fasting is a successful technique for weight reduction for many individuals; but, how exactly does it work?

A decrease in calorie consumption is one of the primary contributors to weight loss that may be accomplished with intermittent fasting. Many individuals find that they are able to consume naturally fewer calories overall when they limit their meals to a set window of time, such as an 8-hour period each day, for example. A decrease in body fat is possible as a result of this calorie shortfall.

However, in addition to these probable processes, intermittent fasting may also be responsible for the weight reduction benefits that it has. For instance, a number of studies have shown that fasting for shorter periods of time than usual may assist increase insulin sensitivity. This, in turn, can lead to better glucose metabolism and a decrease in fat accumulation. In addition, research suggests that intermittent fasting may raise levels of human growth hormone, a hormone that plays a role in both fats burning and the building of lean muscle.

The function of the microbiome as a determinant in weight reduction and metabolism is yet another essential consideration. The term "microbiome" refers to the trillions of different kinds of bacteria that reside in and on the human body, most notably in the digestive tract. These microbes are essential for a number of bodily processes, including digestion, the absorption of nutrients, and immune system function, amongst others.

There is evidence from certain studies that intermittent fasting may help maintain a healthy gut microbiome by lowering inflammation and enhancing the variety and equilibrium of the bacteria that live in the gut. This, in turn, may aid improve overall metabolic health and promote weight reduction efforts.

It is essential to keep in mind that reducing one's body fat and boosting one's metabolism are both intricate processes that are affected by a variety of variables in addition to one's calorie consumption and level of energy expenditure. For instance, the regulation of one's weight and the maintenance of metabolic health may be influenced by one's genes, hormones, and the surrounding environment.

In addition, despite the fact that intermittent fasting has been shown to be a successful technique for weight reduction for many individuals, it may not be suitable for everyone. When beginning a regimen of intermittent fasting, it is possible for some individuals to have undesirable side effects such as headaches, lethargy, or difficulties focusing at the beginning stages of the regimen. In addition, those who have certain medical issues or dietary requirements may need to make adjustments to the intermittent fasting method or completely avoid it.

It is also crucial to highlight that the only way to assess health is by weight reduction and that other aspects, such as the general quality of one's food, the amount of physical exercise one gets, and the ability to manage one's stress, are just as important for one's overall health and well-being.

Even though the science behind weight loss and metabolism is complicated, there is mounting evidence to suggest that intermittent fasting may be a safe and effective strategy for promoting weight loss and improving metabolic health for a large number of people. This is despite the fact that the science behind weight loss and metabolism is complex. However, it is vital to approach intermittent fasting carefully, just as it is necessary to approach any dietary intervention and to speak with a healthcare expert before making substantial changes to your diet or lifestyle before making any dietary or lifestyle changes.

Overall, while the specific mechanisms that are responsible for the weight loss effects of intermittent fasting are still being researched, there is growing evidence to suggest that intermittent fasting may be an effective and sustainable weight loss strategy for many people. This is despite the fact that the exact mechanisms that are responsible for the weight loss effects of intermittent fasting are still being studied. However, it is vital to approach intermittent fasting carefully, just as it is necessary to approach any dietary intervention and to speak with a healthcare expert before making substantial changes to your diet or lifestyle before making any dietary or lifestyle changes.

The Effects of Periodic Fasting on the Aging Process and the Length of One's Life

Research has also been conducted to investigate the possible implications that intermittent fasting may have on aging and lifespan. There is accumulating evidence to indicate that intermittent fasting may have some anti-aging advantages, despite the fact that research in this field is still in its early stages.

As was mentioned previously, the function that intermittent fasting plays in boosting autophagy may be one of the probable mechanisms that underlie the anti-aging benefits of the practice. Through the process of autophagy, damaged and malfunctioning cells, which may build up over time and contribute to the aging process, are removed from the body. Some experts think that we may be able to slow down the aging process and improve lifespan by activating a mechanism called autophagy. This might be accomplished by treatments such as intermittent fasting.

The capacity of intermittent fasting to lower inflammation is another possible reason underlying the anti-aging benefits of this kind of eating pattern. Some studies have shown that intermittent fasting may help decrease inflammation in the body, which is important since chronic inflammation is a critical factor in the development of many age-related disorders.

It is important to keep in mind that although intermittent fasting may have some possible anti-aging advantages, it is not a magic bullet or a promise that one will live for a longer period of time. A person's genes, as well as their surroundings and the choices they make in their daily lives, all play a part in how quickly they age and how long they live.

In addition, while the effects of intermittent fasting on aging and lifespan in humans have been investigated in animal models and in certain studies including people, a greater amount of study is required to completely grasp the topic. It is crucial to highlight that the best fasting regimen for promoting longevity is not yet evident and may vary based on individual characteristics such as age, health condition, and lifestyle choices. It is also important to note that the optimal fasting regimen for promoting longevity is not yet obvious.

In addition, even though there is a growing interest in the potential anti-aging benefits of intermittent fasting, more research is required to fully understand its effects on longevity and to determine the optimal fasting regimen for promoting health and longevity in humans. This is the case even though there is a growing interest in the potential anti-aging benefits of intermittent fasting. In the meantime, it is essential to place emphasis on other aspects of one's lifestyle that are known to promote overall health and well-being. These aspects include engaging in regular physical activity, maintaining a healthy diet, effectively managing stress, and cultivating meaningful social connections.

Additionally, there is some evidence that intermittent fasting might assist enhance metabolic health, which is an important component of both aging and lifespan. Enhancing glucose metabolism, decreasing insulin resistance, and fostering healthy microbiota in the gut might all lead to improved general health and a longer lifespan.

Although further study is required to properly understand the effects of intermittent fasting on aging and lifespan, the information that is now available shows that intermittent fasting may have some advantages related to anti-aging. However, it is essential to approach any dietary intervention with caution, and prior to making any substantial changes to either your diet or your lifestyle, you should discuss your plans with a healthcare professional. In addition, it is essential to keep in mind that the processes of aging and living for a long time are both intricate phenomena that are affected by a variety of elements in addition to one's food and way of life.

The Effects of Periodic Fasting on the Health of the Brain and Its Capacity for Cognitive Function

Intermittent fasting has been examined for its influence on brain health and cognitive function in addition to its possible implications on weight reduction, metabolism, and the aging process. There is accumulating evidence to show that intermittent fasting may have some cognitive advantages, especially in terms of boosting brain function and lowering the risk of age-related cognitive decline.

The capacity of intermittent fasting to encourage the formation of new nerve cells in the brain, a process known as neurogenesis, is one of the probable mechanisms that might be behind the cognitive advantages of intermittent fasting. It is well-accepted that neurogenesis plays a crucial part in the processes of learning and memory, and a number of studies point to the possibility that intermittent fasting might assist stimulate this process.

The capacity of intermittent fasting to lower oxidative stress and inflammation in the brain is another probable explanation underlying the cognitive advantages of this kind of eating pattern. It is believed that chronic inflammation and oxidative stress play a role in the development of neurodegenerative disorders like Alzheimer's disease. Some research shows that intermittent fasting may help minimize the chance of developing neurodegenerative diseases.

Also, there is some evidence that intermittent fasting may increase glucose metabolism as well as insulin sensitivity, both of which are critical components of optimal brain health and cognitive performance. It is possible that intermittent fasting might help lower the risk of cognitive decline and enhance general brain function. This is achieved by improving certain metabolic indicators.

Although further study is required to completely understand the influence that intermittent fasting has on brain health and cognitive performance, the information that is now available shows that intermittent fasting may have some beneficial effects on cognitive function. However, it is essential to approach any dietary intervention with caution, and prior to making any substantial changes to either your diet or your lifestyle, you should discuss your plans with a healthcare professional. In addition, the maintenance of good brain health and cognitive performance depends on a number of other lifestyle variables, including regular physical exercise, stress management, and social interactions.

Some research has been conducted to determine whether or not intermittent fasting has any positive effects on cognitive performance. Research that was conducted on rats and published in the Journal of Molecular Neuroscience discovered that intermittent fasting increased the animals' ability to acquire and remember spatial information. Another research that was published in the Journal of Neuroscience Research discovered that mice who were subjected to intermittent fasting had significant improvements in their cognitive performance and a reduction in the amount of oxidative stress they experienced.

There have been a number of studies in humans that point to the possibility that intermittent fasting has positive effects on cognitive performance. Those older persons who participated in intermittent fasting had greater cognitive performance than those who did not participate in the practice, according to the findings of research that was published in the Journal of Nutrition, Health, and

Aging. Another research that was published in the International Journal of Obesity indicated that obese persons who followed intermittent fasting experienced improvements in their cognitive function as well as their mood.

Although the information that is now available shows that intermittent fasting may have some cognitive advantages, it is essential to keep in mind that further study is required to completely understand its impact on brain health and cognitive performance in people. In addition, certain people should not participate in intermittent fasting, and it is essential to discuss any new dietary regimen with a qualified medical professional before beginning the process.

It is important to approach any dietary intervention with caution and to focus on other lifestyle factors that are known to promote brain health and cognitive function. These lifestyle factors include regular physical activity, stress management, and social connections. Although intermittent fasting may have some potential cognitive benefits, it is important to approach any dietary intervention with caution.

CHAPTER THREE

Different Approaches to Intermittent Fasting

There is no one "right" way to carry out the practice of intermittent fasting since there are many distinct methods available. The strategy that is most suitable for you may be determined by your unique requirements, way of life, and personal preferences. The following is a list of some of the more typical ways to use intermittent fasting:

- Time-restricted feeding (TRF)
- Alternate-day fasting (ADF)
- 5:2 fasting
- Eat-stop-eat
- Modified fasting
- Spontaneous meal skipping

It is essential to keep in mind that not all of these strategies are going to work for everyone all of the time. Some people, such as those who have specific medical issues or who are pregnant or nursing, may find that fasting every other day is difficult or even risky to do. One example is those who are unable to breastfeed or who are pregnant. It is always a good idea to talk with a healthcare professional before beginning any new dietary regimen, particularly if you have underlying health concerns. In particular, if you have diabetes, it is very important to contact a healthcare expert.

In addition, it is essential to ensure that throughout the eating times, the emphasis is on consuming meals that are high in nutrients and that are unprocessed rather than stuffing oneself with junk food or processed foods. Instead of focusing just on reducing one's calorie intake or decreasing body weight, the objective of intermittent fasting should be to promote overall health and well-being instead.

Time-Restricted Feeding

The method of intermittent fasting known as time-restricted feeding (TRF) requires participants to restrict the daily window of time in which they are allowed to consume food. This strategy calls for abstaining from food for a period of at least 12 hours, followed by a period of eating during the remaining 12 hours of the day. However, some individuals may opt to increase the amount of time spent fasting each day to 14, 16, or even 18 hours.

TRF may be carried out in a number of distinct ways. One strategy that is often used is to have your first meal of the day later in the day, say at ten in the morning, and then have your final meal of the day earlier, say at six in the evening. This results in an eating window of eight hours and a fasting window of sixteen hours. Some individuals prefer to eat just two meals per day, while others choose to eat three meals per day or multiple smaller meals spread out throughout the day. Others still choose to snack throughout the day.

It has been shown that TRF may provide a number of positive health effects. One of the most important advantages is that it can assist in the regulation of circadian rhythms. Circadian rhythms are internal biological rhythms that regulate a wide variety of physiological processes, such as the production of hormones and the rate at which one's metabolism operates while sleeping. It has been shown that TRF may enhance circadian rhythms, which in turn can have a beneficial effect on one's general health.

It has also been shown that TRF may increase insulin sensitivity, which refers to the capacity of the body to make efficient use of insulin in order to manage blood sugar levels. People who struggle with insulin resistance or type 2 diabetes may benefit significantly from this in particular. In addition to this, there is evidence that TRF may assist with weight reduction and improve cardiovascular health indices such as blood pressure and cholesterol levels.

It is essential to keep in mind that TRF may not be suitable for everyone, especially those who suffer from certain medical disorders, are pregnant or nursing, or have certain other life circumstances. In addition, it is essential to ensure that throughout the eating times, the emphasis is on consuming meals that are high in nutrients and that are unprocessed rather than stuffing oneself with junk food or processed foods. Instead of focusing on weight loss or calorie restriction as the primary objective of TRF, the organization needs to have as its primary mission the promotion of general health and well-being.

Although the fasting method known as time-restricted feeding, or TRF, may be an efficient method for intermittent fasting, it is not the only way to fast. The practice of fasting for a complete 24 hours every other day, known as alternate-day fasting, may appeal more to some individuals. Others may like the 5:2 diet, which consists of eating regularly for five days out of the week and then reducing the number of calories consumed to between 500 and 600 per day for two days that are not consecutive.

Alternate-day fasting (ADF)

Alternate day fasting, often known as ADF, is a kind of intermittent fasting that includes alternating days of regular eating with days of fasting. The goal of this method is to reduce overall caloric intake. During the days of the fast, one's caloric intake is limited to 25% of their regular level, which is normally somewhere around 500 calories for women and 600 calories for men. People are permitted to eat regularly on the days when they are not fasting.

It has been shown that ADF may have a number of beneficial effects on one's health. According to the findings of many studies, consuming ADF may result in a decrease in body fat as well as an increase in muscle mass, both of which contribute to better body composition. It has also been shown that consumption of ADF may benefit cardiovascular health by lowering blood pressure, cholesterol levels, and inflammatory markers.

One possible benefit of alternate day fasting (ADF) over other kinds of intermittent fasting is that it allows for regular eating on non-fasting days, which may make it more manageable for certain individuals. Other forms of intermittent fasting do not allow for normal eating on non-fasting days. On the other hand, some individuals could find it difficult to keep to the stringent calorie limitations on fasting days, especially over the course of a longer period of time.

It is essential to keep in mind that the ADF may not be the right choice for everyone. During fasting days, those who have certain medical disorders, such as diabetes, may need to keep a careful eye on their blood sugar levels in order to prevent hypoglycemia from occurring. In addition, there is a possibility that ADF is not appropriate for women who are pregnant or nursing, as well as for persons who have a history of eating disorders.

When engaging in any kind of intermittent fasting, it is essential to concentrate your eating sessions on the consumption of whole foods that are rich in nutrients in order to provide your body with the nutrition it requires. In addition, it is essential to consume a large amount of water and maintain a state of hydration, especially on days when one is fasting. You may assess whether or not the ADF is a method that is secure and acceptable for you by having a conversation with a healthcare physician or a trained dietitian.

Some researchers have pointed to the possibility that ADF may also be beneficial to the health of the brain. According to the findings of one research conducted on mice, the administration of ADF boosted cognitive performance and stimulated the creation of new neurons in the hippocampus. This region of the brain is responsible for learning and memory. In yet another study involving humans, researchers discovered that ADF was connected with increased executive function. Executive function refers to activities such as planning, decision-making, and working memory.

Additionally, there is a possibility that ADF might help individuals who are coping with specific medical situations. According to the findings of one research, ADF alleviated symptoms in persons who suffered from asthma, while another study discovered that ADF decreased symptoms and enhanced quality of life in people who suffered from rheumatoid arthritis.

On the other hand, it is essential to point out that further study is required in order to get a complete understanding of the possible advantages and hazards of ADF. In addition, some individuals may discover that adhering to the ADF for an extended period of time is difficult for them, especially if they have a history of eating disorders.

It is crucial to approach ADF with caution and to speak with a healthcare physician or certified dietitian before beginning, just as it is necessary to do so with any other kind of intermittent fasting. They will be able to advise you on how to approach fasting days to ensure that you are achieving your nutritional requirements and will be able to assist you to assess whether or not ADF is a method that is safe and suitable for you.

5:2 Abstinence and Fasting

The 5:2 diet is another kind of intermittent fasting that entails eating normally for five days of the week and limiting calorie intake to between 500 and 600 calories for two days of the week that are not consecutive. This helps dieters lose weight by reducing their overall calorie consumption. People who are participating in the fasting days may choose to consume one or two smaller meals or snacks spaced throughout the day rather than a single bigger meal during this time period.

It has been shown that following the 5:2 diet may have various positive effects on one's health. According to a number of studies, it may result in a loss in body weight, a decrease in total body fat, and an increase in insulin sensitivity. The diet may also have positive effects on cardiovascular health, such as lower risks of cardiovascular disease and improvements in blood pressure, cholesterol levels, and inflammatory indicators.

When compared to other types of intermittent fasting, the 5:2 diet has the potential benefit of allowing for more flexibility and less stringent calorie tracking on non-fasting days. This is one of the possible advantages of the diet. On the other hand, some individuals can find it difficult to adhere to the stringent calorie limitations that are imposed on fasting days.

When engaging in any kind of intermittent fasting, it is essential to concentrate your eating sessions on the consumption of whole foods that are rich in nutrients in order to provide your body with the nutrition it requires. In addition, it is essential to consume a large amount of water and maintain a state of hydration, especially on days when one is fasting. If you are unsure whether or not the 5:2 diet is a healthy and viable option for you, consulting with a certified dietitian or a healthcare practitioner may help you make this determination.

One of the possible drawbacks of the 5:2 diet is that it isn't recommended for persons who are at risk of hypoglycemia or who have a history of disordered eating. This is because the 5:2 diet restricts carbohydrate consumption to every other day. In addition, some individuals may have a hard time adhering to the stringent calorie limitations that are imposed during fasting days, which may cause them to overeat or binge eat on days when they are not required to fast.

In addition, it is essential to keep in mind that the 5:2 diet may not be suitable for everyone. On days when they are fasting, those who have certain medical problems, such as diabetes, may need to change the dosages of their medications or insulin in order to prevent hypoglycemia. Without the supervision of a qualified medical professional, women who are pregnant or nursing, children, and adolescents should not participate in intermittent fasting.

It is essential to approach the 5:2 diet with prudence and to have a discussion with a healthcare physician or trained dietitian before beginning the diet, as is the case with any other kind of intermittent fasting. They will be able to assist you in determining whether or not the 5:2 diet is a strategy that is secure and suitable for you. Additionally, they will be able to provide assistance on how to handle fasting days to ensure that you are achieving your nutritional requirements.

Spontaneous Meal Skipping

The practice of missing meals on an ad hoc basis in order to achieve the health benefits of intermittent fasting is known as spontaneous meal skipping. Because it focuses on paying attention to your body's hunger and satiety signals to decide when you should eat, this method is also known as "listen-to-your-body" fasting or "listen-to-your-body" fasting.

There are no predetermined timetables or regulations regarding the times at which one must eat or not eat while engaging in spontaneous meal skipping. Instead, you eat just when you're famished and skip meals when you're not in need of nourishment. This method can be especially useful for people who prefer a more flexible approach to fast, as it enables greater variation in the timing of meals and can be adapted to fit a variety of lifestyles and schedules. As a result, it can be especially beneficial for people who prefer a more flexible approach to fasting.

According to research, skipping meals on purpose may be an effective strategy for promoting weight reduction and improving metabolic health. This is because it helps to minimize the number of calories consumed and improves the body's sensitivity to insulin. However, it is essential to keep in mind that this strategy may not be suitable for everyone, particularly those who suffer from certain medical issues, who are pregnant or nursing, or who are of a certain age.

If skipping meals on an impromptu basis is something you're interested in doing, it's crucial to do so in a careful and deliberate manner from the beginning. Pay attention to the signals that your body sends you about hunger and fullness, and make sure that your food is well-balanced and contains all of the nutrients that your body requires. In addition, be ready to make any necessary adjustments to your strategy, and if you have any concerns about your current state of health or nutrition, seek the advice of a certified dietitian or a healthcare specialist who specializes in nutrition.

People who are new to the practice of fasting may find that missing meals on an impromptu basis is a helpful alternative since it gives them a taste of what it is like to go without eating without requiring them to adhere to a regimented timetable or specific method of fasting. People who are already acquainted with fasting and wish to add a more flexible approach to their practice may also find it to be a helpful tool.

One possible benefit of missing meals on an impromptu basis is that, in comparison to other methods of fasting, it enables a higher degree of flexibility and adaptation. This can be especially helpful for people who have busy schedules or unpredictable lifestyles because it enables them to skip meals when they need to without having to worry about sticking to a set schedule. This can be especially beneficial for people who have busy schedules or unpredictable lifestyles.

However, it is essential to keep in mind that missing a meal on the spur of the moment may not be ideal for everyone. For instance, in order to properly manage their health, those who suffer from certain medical illnesses, such as diabetes or eating disorders, may be required to adhere to a more regimented method of fasting than healthy individuals. Even if you often go without food, you still need to make sure that you are providing your body with all of the nutrients it requires. This is true even if you are missing meals.

There are a few things you can take to guarantee that you are spontaneously skipping meals in a way that is both safe and beneficial to your health if you are contemplating giving it a try. First, it is important to pay attention to the signals of hunger and satiety that your body sends you and to make an effort to eat only when you are hungry and to stop eating when you are no longer hungry. Even if you are skipping meals sometimes, you should still make it a priority to have a healthy, well-rounded diet that is rich in a variety of foods, such as fruits, vegetables, whole grains, and lean sources of protein.

In general, missing meals on an impromptu basis might be an excellent choice for those who are seeking a kind of fasting that allows for more flexibility. However, it is crucial to approach it carefully and with purpose, and if you have any concerns about your health or nutritional status, you should seek counsel from a healthcare physician or qualified dietitian.

Combining Fasting with Other Diets to Achieve Your Health Goals

It is possible to combine intermittent fasting with several other dietary practices in order to further boost its effects or to meet certain health objectives. Combining intermittent fasting with a ketogenic diet, commonly known as a low-carbohydrate, high-fat diet, is a popular choice among those who want to lose weight. Each of these treatments has been found to increase weight reduction, improve insulin sensitivity, and decrease inflammation; thus, it is believed that this combination will boost the effects of both of these approaches.

A diet that is mostly composed of plant foods is yet another method of eating that may be paired with intermittent fasting. Plant-based diets have been linked to a lower risk of chronic illnesses such as heart disease and diabetes. Plant-based diets are abundant in fiber, vitamins, and minerals. A plant-based diet, when paired with intermittent fasting, may further boost the advantages of both techniques.

Combining intermittent fasting with activities such as calorie counting or monitoring macronutrient intake is one way to improve the likelihood that you will provide your body with the essential nutrition it requires during meal windows. This may be of utmost significance if you are striving to accomplish certain health objectives, such as increasing your muscle mass or decreasing your body fat percentage.

Before combining intermittent fasting with other dietary approaches, it is essential to discuss the matter with a healthcare professional or a qualified dietitian, as is the case with any nutritional method. They will be able to assist you in determining if the combination is safe and suitable for you, and they will also be able to provide assistance about how to properly balance your nutrient intake in order to satisfy your individual requirements.

Although it may be helpful to combine fasting with other dietary techniques, it is crucial to keep in mind that not all dietary approaches are suitable for use in conjunction with fasting. For instance, eating a diet that is heavy in carbohydrates may lead to spikes and falls in blood sugar levels, which can be challenging to regulate during times of fasting. In a similar vein, if you eat a diet that is heavy in processed foods or sugar, it may be difficult to achieve your fasting objectives, and it may also hinder your attempts to lose weight.

When combining intermittent fasting with other types of diets, it is essential to pay attention to the requirements of your body and modify your strategy according to those requirements. For instance, if you're experiencing symptoms such as weariness or lightheadedness while you're fasting, it's possible that you need to make adjustments to either your nutritional intake or your fasting schedule. In addition, if you are not getting the results you want from the combination of fasting and dieting that you are doing, it is possible that you will need to make some adjustments to your strategy or seek the advice of a healthcare professional or a registered dietitian in order to receive additional direction.

In the end, the most important thing to keep in mind when attempting to combine intermittent fasting with other diets is to go into it with an open mind, a lot of patience, and a willingness to explore. It is feasible to obtain major health advantages and to build a lifestyle that is both healthy and sustainable if the appropriate strategy is taken.

CHAPTER FOUR

Implementing Intermittent Fasting into Your Lifestyle

If you want to enhance your health and well-being, including intermittent fasting in your lifestyle may be an excellent option for you. However, it is essential to take a deliberate and measured approach to it, as well as to adapt your strategy to the specific requirements and preferences of the person you are working with.

How to Get Started with the Health Benefits of Intermittent Fasting

Choose a method of fasting that is appropriate for you: There is a wide variety of fasting protocols available; thus, it is essential to pick one that is suitable for your lifestyle as well as your tastes. The 5:2 diet, time-restricted eating, and alternate-day fasting are all popular choices among those looking to lose weight. Experiment with a variety of methods until you discover one that you can maintain and is pleasurable for you.

Start slowly: If you've never tried fasting before, it's important to take it easy at first and work your way up to longer periods without eating. As an example, you may start by missing breakfast a few times a week, and then progressively increase the number of days that you go without eating.

Stay Hydrated: Drink lots of water and other hydrating drinks throughout your fasting times to keep hydrated and help lessen sensations of hunger. It is vital to drink enough water and other hydrating beverages during your fasting intervals. You may also help fend off hunger by drinking liquids like tea, coffee, and other drinks that are low in calories.

Plan Your Meals: When you're not fasting, it's crucial to consume a balanced diet that contains lots of whole foods that are high in nutrients. It's also important to plan your meals. For the sake of your health and well-being, it is important to prepare your meals in advance and check that you are receiving an adequate amount of protein, healthy fats, and complex carbs.

Pay attention to your body: While fasting may be an effective method for improving your health, you must pay attention to your body and make any necessary adjustments to your strategy. During your fasting times, if you notice that you are feeling excessively hungry, exhausted, or ill, this may be a clue that you need to make adjustments to your fasting protocol or seek the advice of a healthcare practitioner.

Be patient and persistent: Just like any other adjustment to your lifestyle, intermittent fasting requires you to be patient and consistent to experience benefits. Continue doing what you're doing, be patient with yourself, and keep in mind that making little, step-by-step adjustments throughout some time may lead to significant gains in your health and well-being.

Overall, making intermittent fasting a regular part of your lifestyle may be a potent approach to enhance both your health and your overall well-being. You may build a sustainable and fun approach to fasting that promotes your health and happiness by beginning gently, planning your meals, and listening to your body. This will help you establish a sustainable and happy approach to fasting.

How to Get Ready for Fasting Periods That Are Spaced Apart

It is necessary to prepare yourself psychologically as well as physically before beginning intermittent fasting to increase the likelihood that you will have a positive experience with the practice. Here are some suggestions to assist you in getting ready:

Check with your healthcare provider: It is always a good idea to talk with your doctor before beginning any new diet or fitness routine, but this is particularly important to do if you already suffer from any pre-existing medical concerns.

Determine the best timetable for your fasting: There is a wide variety of fasting schedules available to select from; thus, it is essential to pick the one that is most suitable for you in terms of your lifestyle. When choosing a fasting plan, it is important to take into consideration your normal routine, including your job schedule and any other social obligations.

Begin with a low gear: If you are new to the practice of fasting, it is recommended that you begin slowly and gradually build up to fasting for extended periods. Start with a fast that lasts for 12 hours, and then progressively extend it by an additional hour or two every few days until you reach the length of time that you want it to last.

Prepare your meals in advance: When you're not fasting, it's essential to prepare your meals in advance to ensure that you consume a nutritious and well-balanced diet. Put your emphasis on consuming entire meals that are high in nutrients, such as fruits, vegetables, lean meats, and healthy fats.

Maintaining enough hydration: is of the utmost importance while engaging in any kind of fasting. Consume a lot of water, and if you feel like it, try adding some electrolytes to it. This will assist your body restore its supplies.

Take steps to control your stress: Because fasting may be taxing on your body, you must take steps to regulate your stress levels while you are engaging in this practice. Try doing some stress-relieving activities like yoga, meditation, or just taking some slow, deep breaths.

Determine the reasons you have chosen to fast: Discovering why you want to give intermittent fasting a go might be beneficial to your experience with the practice. Having a clear grasp of your objectives may help motivate you and keep you on track, regardless of whether you want to lose weight, boost your energy levels, or get any of the other potential health advantages.

Find a support system: When beginning a new diet or making other significant changes to one's lifestyle, it may be tremendously beneficial to have the support of friends, family, or a community of people who share similar values. If you want to interact with other people who are going through a journey similar to yours, you can think about joining an online forum or a social media group that is devoted to intermittent fasting.

Be flexible: While you must adhere to your fasting schedule as strictly as is humanly feasible, it is also essential that you maintain some degree of adaptability when circumstances so require it. Don't be too harsh on yourself if you have a social event or another engagement that falls outside of your fasting period. Just make sure that you give your fasting routine your very best effort to get the finest results possible.

Maintain a record of your accomplishments: Keeping a record of your accomplishments may be an effective tool for maintaining your motivation and ensuring that you stay on course. You may want to maintain a notebook in which you record your fasting schedule, the meals you eat, and any changes in your body or energy levels that you see.

Get adequate sleep: Getting a sufficient amount of sleep is necessary for one's health in general, but it is of utmost significance during times of fasting. Aim for seven to eight hours of sleep every night to assist and support the natural processes that occur in your body.

You may assist guarantee that you are well-prepared for the journey of intermittent fasting by putting into practice the advice that has been provided here. Always keep in mind the importance of having patience with yourself and dealing with difficulties one day at a time. After some time has passed, you will discover that fasting is becoming simpler and more natural for you, and you will start to experience the myriad of positive health effects that are associated with continuing this practice.

Managing Hunger and Cravings

When you first start practicing intermittent fasting, it might be difficult to keep your hunger and desires under control, particularly in the beginning. The following is a list of advice that will help you cope with hunger and cravings:

Consuming enough water: may assist in reducing feelings of hunger and helping you feel fuller after eating. Aim to consume between 8 and 10 glasses of water every single day.

Consume some coffee or tea: Both coffee and tea have been shown to reduce hunger and speed up the metabolism. Just make sure that neither sugar nor creamer is added to your beverage of choice (coffee or tea).

Consume foods that are rich in fiber: Consuming foods that are high in fiber, such as fruits, vegetables, and grains that are whole, may help you feel full and satisfied for extended periods.

Consume meals that are high in protein: Protein has been shown to help lessen sensations of hunger while simultaneously increasing feelings of fullness. Meat, fish, and poultry, as well as eggs, beans, and lentils, are all excellent sources of protein.

Make a plan for your meals: Making a meal plan in advance will assist you in maintaining your fasting schedule and lessen the risk that you will consume an excessive amount of food.

Maintain your busy schedule; this will make it less likely that you will think about eating. Find ways to keep yourself engaged during the time that you are not eating, such as by reading, engaging in physical activity, or hanging out with friends.

Take steps to manage your stress; it may be the cause of your appetite and desires. Find healthy strategies to deal with your stress, such as yoga, meditation, or workouts that require deep breathing.

Get adequate sleep; not getting enough sleep may cause hormones that control hunger and fullness to become disrupted, which can lead to an increased appetite and increased desire for unhealthy foods. Aim to obtain 7-8 hours of sleep every night.

Don't skip meals: It is not a good idea to miss meals since doing so might make you hungrier and increase the probability that you will overeat at a later time. Maintain a regular eating schedule and avoid skipping any of your meals.

Try these foods that are low in calories: If you find that you are becoming hungry in between meals, consider munching on some raw veggies or a piece of fruit for a snack that is low in calories.

Chew gum: Chewing gum may help minimize sensations of hunger and also make it easier to avoid snacking on unhealthy foods when you're hungry.

Eat with awareness and presence: When you do eat, pay attention to what you are eating and be present at the moment. Take your time and savor each morsel when you consume food. This may make you feel more satiated and lower the probability that you will eat more than you need to.

Allow for flexibility: Although maintaining your fasting schedule is very essential, it is also acceptable to allow yourself some wiggle room. Do not let the fact that you will need to change your eating routine to accommodate a certain event or occasion cause you concern. Simply go back on course as soon as you can.

Always keep in mind that it is important to pay attention to your body and provide it with the nourishment it requires. If you are fasting and find that you are feeling excessively hungry or have severe desires, this may be an indication that you need to tweak the timing of your fast or make some adjustments to the foods that you eat.

What to Consume for Food and Drink Throughout the Fasting Period

During the time that you are supposed to be fasting, you must abstain from eating anything that contains calories or anything else that can cause you to break your fast. This includes consumable items in solid form, drinks with calorie content, and even specific supplements with calorie content.

Nevertheless, it is essential to maintain an adequate level of hydration during the duration of fasting. You don't need any sugar or milk to enjoy beverages such as water, sparkling water, or herbal tea.

Because it has such a low-calorie content, black coffee is permitted to be consumed throughout the time of fasting.

During the period when they are required to abstain from eating and drinking, some individuals discover that drinking water that has been electrolyte-enhanced or swallowing a tiny quantity of sea salt mixed with water will assist them in maintaining their levels of hydration and vitality.

It is essential to keep in mind that the kind of food you consume during the eating window may also have a big effect on your efforts to improve your health and achieve your desired weight reduction. In general, it is suggested that one consume whole foods that are high in nutritional density and abundant in fiber, protein, and healthy fats.

The following are some selections that are both nutritious and delicious: leafy greens, vegetables, and fruits; lean meats such as chicken, fish, and tofu; whole grains such as brown rice and quinoa; nuts, seeds, and healthy oils such as olive oil and avocado oil, stay away from processed meals, sugary beverages, and snacks as much as possible since they may trigger cravings and produce increases in blood sugar.

When determining what to eat and drink within your eating window, here are some additional considerations to take into account:

Take into consideration the sizes of the portions: The fact that you are permitted to eat within the allotted time does not imply that you should stuff yourself silly with food. Pay attention to the amounts of the portions you are served, and eat until you are satisfied but not too full.

Consume your food cautiously and slowly: Spend some time appreciating the flavor of the food you're eating and paying attention to how it makes you feel after eating it. Eating slowly may help you become more attuned to your body's signals of hunger and fullness, hence reducing the likelihood that you will consume an excessive amount of food.

Concentrate on the protein: Consuming protein throughout your allotted meal time might help you feel fuller for a longer period and may assist in the maintenance of your muscle mass.

Don't forget about fiber: Fiber plays a key role in digestive health and may also assist in maintaining a sensation of fullness in the body. Make it a priority to load up on fruits, veggies, whole grains, and legumes whenever you sit down to eat.

Consider the preparation of meals: It might be simpler to keep to your eating plan and avoid making unhealthy choices if you plan and prepare your meals in advance. Planning and preparing your meals in advance can assist.

Stay hydrated: Consuming a lot of water and other liquids that are low in calories will help you feel full longer and keep your body hydrated.

Keep in mind that the most essential step is to choose a diet that is compatible with your way of life and can help you achieve your goals. Consider consulting with a trained dietitian if you are having problems determining what foods and beverages to consume throughout your eating window. A registered dietitian can give individualized suggestions that are based on the client's specific requirements and objectives.

How to Break the Fast Without Risking Your Health

Observing proper protocol when you break your fast is an essential component of practicing intermittent fasting. The following are some considerations to bear in mind:

To get started, have a light meal: If you have gone for a long time without eating, the first meal you consume after that should be somewhat light so as not to tax your digestive system too quickly. A light lunch that is well-balanced and contains protein, healthy fats, and complex carbs is sometimes a smart place to start when trying to lose weight.

Pick meals high in nutrients: When it's time to break your fast, pick foods that are high in nutrients and will offer your body the fuel it needs to function properly. Green leafy vegetables, vegetables in general, fruits, nuts, seeds, and whole grains are some examples.

Steer clear of processed foods: Consuming processed meals and beverages that are high in sugar may put a strain on your digestive system and lead to an increase in your blood sugar levels. When breaking your fast, it is in your best interest to steer clear of these categories of foods.

Hydrate: It is essential to replenish the body's fluids after it has been deprived of them for some time. Consume a lot of water and other fluids that may help you stay hydrated, such as herbal tea, coconut water, or bone broth.

Pay attention to your bodily cues: After you have broken your fast, pay attention to how your body feels in general. If you feel any pain, bloating, or indigestion, make a mental note of the things that you may be eating that are contributing to the issue and alter your diet appropriately.

Keep in mind that breaking your fast healthily and safely is as vital as the fast itself. Taking the time to slowly reintroduce food to your body after a period of intermittent fasting may help you avoid pain and enable you to get the most out of the health advantages of the practice.

Overcoming Obstacles That Are Often Encountered

Some individuals may find it difficult, particularly in the beginning, to adhere to an intermittent fasting schedule. The following is a list of typical difficulties that individuals confront, along with suggestions for overcoming them:

Hunger: Feeling hungry is a frequent occurrence while beginning intermittent fasting, however, most people find that their hunger disappears after a few days of practicing the technique. Drinking enough fluids, such as water, tea, or coffee, will help you feel filled for longer, which can be helpful when trying to control hunger. Consuming meals that are rich in protein throughout your eating window might also assist in reducing feelings of hunger.

Cravings: It may be challenging to resist cravings for certain meals, particularly when one is in the midst of a period of fasting. Distracting oneself from other activities, such as working out, meditating, or reading is one strategy for overcoming urges to indulge in unhealthy behaviors. You may also make a meal plan in advance and have some nutritious snacks on hand to consume during the time that you are allowed to eat to assist fulfill cravings.

Social Pressure: When you are around by others who are eating, such as friends or family, it might be difficult to adhere to an intermittent fasting regimen. It may be beneficial to have a conversation with them about your objectives and the reasons you have chosen to fast. You may make it simpler for yourself to keep to your fasting schedule by scheduling social engagements to take place during the time that you are allowed to consume food.

Very Little Energy: During the beginning phases of intermittent fasting, some individuals find that they have less energy than usual. This is normal when your body adjusts to the new pattern of eating that you have been following. A lack of energy may be helped by ensuring that enough rest is obtained and that adequate hydration is maintained throughout the day. Caffeine, which may be found in beverages like coffee and tea, is another way to help improve energy levels.

Plateaus: When following an intermittent fasting regimen for a considerable amount of time, it is possible to reach a point when you no longer notice any effects, which is known as a plateau. This may be because your body has adjusted to the new dietary pattern you've been following. You can get around this by varying the timing of your fasts or ramping up the intensity of your exercises, both of which are options.

Social events: When you're trying to stick to your intermittent fasting routine, it may be challenging to manage social situations like parties and get-togethers. It is vital to prepare ahead and communicate with friends and family about your fasting schedule to prevent circumstances in which you may be tempted to break your fast. This will allow you to avoid situations where you may be tempted to break your fast.

Exercising: Some individuals find that it is difficult to exercise when they are fasting, particularly if they are going for a prolonged amount of time without eating. It is essential to pay attention to what your body is telling you and to modify your workout program accordingly. While some individuals feel that exercising during their eating window is more beneficial, others find that exercising during their fasting time is more beneficial.

Digestive difficulties: While practicing intermittent fasting, some individuals may have digestive issues such as bloating or constipation. Other people may not experience these concerns at all. To maintain good digestion, it is essential to drink lots of water and consume a wide variety of foods that are high in fiber while you are allowed to eat.

Sleep disturbances: While practicing intermittent fasting, some individuals may find that they have trouble sleeping, particularly if they are engaging in a lengthier fast than normal. Avoiding coffee and electronic devices an hour or so before going to bed, as well as committing to a consistent sleep routine, should be high on your list of priorities when it comes to proper sleep hygiene.

Plateaus and setbacks: It is typical to suffer plateaus or setbacks when practicing intermittent fasting, particularly if you are using it as a technique for weight reduction. This is especially true if you are using it as a strategy for losing weight. Even if it appears like you aren't making much progress, it's crucial to keep your motivation up and keep making good choices.

You may improve your chances of having success with intermittent fasting by familiarizing yourself with the most frequent obstacles that arise and putting plans in place to overcome those obstacles.

CHAPTER FIVE

The Future of Intermittent Fasting

In recent years, intermittent fasting has seen a rise in popularity, and this trend will probably continue in the foreseeable future. Ongoing studies are being conducted to investigate the health advantages of intermittent fasting; however, there is still a great deal to understand about the many methods that may be used and how they influence a variety of groups. It is conceivable that new ways to intermittent fasting could arise, or that current techniques will be enhanced or integrated with other dietary treatments to maximize health results. Another possibility is that intermittent fasting will be studied more extensively in the future.

The possibility for individualized intermittent fasting regimens that are adapted to an individual's unique requirements and objectives about their health is one area that is drawing a lot of attention. As the study of nutrigenomics continues to grow, it may become feasible to find genetic markers that can be used to drive the creation of tailored fasting regimens. This would be a significant step forward in the area of nutrigenomics. Additionally, emerging technology such as continuous glucose monitoring and wearable gadgets may make it simpler for individuals to monitor their fasting and eating habits to improve their outcomes. This might be a positive development for people with diabetes. The potential for intermittent fasting to be utilized in concert with other lifestyle therapies such as exercise and stress reduction to enhance the health benefits is another area of study that is currently being conducted. It has been reported by several studies that combining exercise with intermittent fasting may lead to larger changes in body composition and metabolic health than either strategy alone.

In general, it seems that intermittent fasting has a bright future, and it is quite probable that it will continue to be a topic of intense study and development within the fields of nutrition and health. It is possible that when more information is discovered about the processes that underlie its advantages and the appropriate ways for various groups, it will become a more popular and successful tool for enhancing health and avoiding chronic illness.

The Most Recent Studies and Fast-Developing Trends

Research into the practice of intermittent fasting is expanding at a rapid rate, and there are already a large number of studies looking at the possible health advantages of this eating pattern as well as investigating novel variants and procedures.

Ongoing studies are investigating the effects of intermittent fasting on a variety of health issues, including diabetes, cardiovascular disease, and cancer. These studies are part of the current research that is being conducted on intermittent fasting. Emerging trends in intermittent fasting include the use of personalized approaches that take into account individual differences in response to fasting, as well as the utilization of technology and wearable devices to monitor and track fasting periods and meal timing. Personalized approaches have been shown to have a positive impact on health and wellness.

In addition, there is a growing interest in the potential advantages of combining intermittent fasting with other lifestyle treatments like exercising and practicing mindfulness. This interest comes from the fact that such a combination has been shown to have synergistic effects. There has been a recent uptick in the number of healthcare practitioners and wellness coaches who include fasting as a component of their treatment regimens for their patients. This is part of a larger trend toward the integration of fasting into mainstream healthcare and wellness practices.

There is reason to be optimistic about the future of intermittent fasting, as both continuing research and developing trends point to its potential for enhancing health and well-being. However, before beginning a regimen of intermittent fasting, it is important to consult with a healthcare professional, just as it is important to do so before beginning any kind of dietary or lifestyle intervention. This is done to ensure that the regimen is safe and appropriate for the individual's needs and health status. The following are some examples of developing tendencies in the industry:

1. Time-restricted eating, also known as TRF, is becoming more popular as a type of intermittent fasting since it is easier to manage and offers more flexibility. Instead of adhering to rigorous fasting and feeding schedules, TRF entails restricting the amount of time you spend eating each day (usually between 8 and 12 hours) and then fasting for the remaining hours of the day.

2. The possible health advantages of fasting for longer periods are now being researched. Some researchers are researching the impact of extended fasting periods on the body, with early studies revealing encouraging outcomes for inflammation, metabolism, and cellular repair. These periods of fasting may last for up to 48 or even 72 hours.

3. Combination diets that include intermittent fasting as one of many dietary regimens are now being researched for their potential to improve health benefits. For instance, the "ketogenic diet," which is low in carbs and high in fat, may work well in combination with intermittent fasting to help manage blood sugar levels and encourage weight reduction. The ketogenic diet is rich in fat and low in carbohydrates.

4. The effects of intermittent fasting on certain groups, such as athletes, older individuals, and persons with chronic health issues like diabetes or cancer, have been the subject of an increasing number of studies in recent years.

The research suggests that intermittent fasting has significant potential as a tool for improving overall health and wellness, and it is likely that new studies will continue exploring its many applications and benefits in the years to come. Overall, the research suggests that intermittent fasting has significant potential as a tool for improving overall health and wellness.

The Possible Therapeutic Benefits of Periodic Fasting for several Different Health Conditions

It has been discovered that there may be beneficial effects of intermittent fasting on a variety of health issues. While more study has to be done, the following are some of the ailments that might be helped by following an intermittent fasting schedule:

Diabetic Type 2: There is some evidence that intermittent fasting may assist improve blood sugar control as well as insulin sensitivity, both of which are essential components of diabetes management.

Cardiovascular Disease: Intermittent fasting has been demonstrated to help decrease blood pressure, reduce inflammation, and improve cholesterol levels, all of which may lead to a reduced risk of cardiovascular disease. These studies have indicated that intermittent fasting may help lower the risk of cardiovascular disease.

Neurodegenerative Diseases: There is some evidence to suggest that intermittent fasting may help protect against neurodegenerative diseases such as Alzheimer's and Parkinson's by reducing oxidative stress and inflammation in the brain. This is accomplished by restricting a person's caloric intake on alternating days.

Cancer: Intermittent fasting may help prevent cancer by slowing the development and spread of cancer cells, as shown by several scientific research.

Autoimmune Diseases: Intermittent fasting may assist in the reduction of inflammation and the improvement of the function of the immune system. As a result, individuals who suffer from autoimmune diseases such as rheumatoid arthritis and multiple sclerosis may benefit from the practice of intermittent fasting.

It is crucial to emphasize that further study is required in these areas and that intermittent fasting should not be used as a substitute for medical treatment or advice from a qualified medical professional.

The Importance of Periodic Fasting in the Field of Preventative Medicine

There is growing evidence that intermittent fasting may help prevent or improve a broad variety of health issues, including type 2 diabetes, cardiovascular disease, obesity, and some forms of cancer. These studies have shown encouraging outcomes. Intermittent fasting has been shown to enhance general health, as well as minimize the chance of acquiring chronic illnesses such as diabetes and cardiovascular disease. This is accomplished through lowering insulin resistance, normalizing blood sugar levels, and lowering inflammation.

In addition, research has shown that intermittent fasting may have anti-aging benefits by enhancing the processes of cellular repair and boosting the development of new cells. Additionally, it may enhance cognitive performance and protect against neurodegenerative disorders such as Parkinson's disease and Alzheimer's disease.

To have a complete understanding of the possible health advantages of intermittent fasting and how it may be employed in preventative medicine, further study is required. However, the data available at this time shows that using intermittent fasting as part of a healthy lifestyle may be an effective method to lower the risk of developing chronic illnesses and enhance general health.

CONCLUSION

It has been shown that a strategy known as intermittent fasting may help people lose weight, improve their metabolic health, and lower their chance of developing chronic illnesses. Enhancements in brain function, increased lifespan, and general well-being are additional potential outcomes of this practice. However, intermittent fasting is not a panacea, and it may not be appropriate for those who have certain medical conditions. Before beginning a new diet or making significant changes to your lifestyle, it is essential to discuss your plans with a qualified medical practitioner. This is particularly important if you are already taking medication or suffer from a medical condition. Additionally, it is essential to approach the practice of intermittent fasting with a flexible mentality and to pay attention to the requirements of your body. It is vital to approach intermittent fasting with prudence and make educated choices based on your unique requirements and objectives, but overall, it may be a beneficial tool for enhancing health and well-being.

Before beginning any new eating plan or fitness routine, it is critical to discuss the changes with a qualified medical practitioner. Especially if you have any underlying medical concerns, your physician will be able to assist you in determining whether or not intermittent fasting is safe and acceptable for you to engage in.

When you have been given the all-clear from your doctor, the next step is to choose an intermittent fasting regimen that will be most beneficial to you in light of your lifestyle. As was said previously, there are several ways to implement intermittent fasting; thus, it is essential to pick a method that is suited to both your requirements and preferences. It may take some time for your body to adapt when you first begin intermittent fasting. Therefore, it is better to start cautiously, such as by restricting the amount of time you spend eating, and gradually increasing the amount of time you spend fasting over time. In addition, ensure that you drink enough water during the fasting time, and break your fast with meals that are rich in nutrients to meet the requirements of your body.

It is important to keep in mind that intermittent fasting is not a one-size-fits-all method and that what is successful for one person may not be successful for another. It is essential to pay attention to what your body is telling you and to make necessary changes. The keys to success are patience and tenacity, and it could take some time before you get the results you want.

In conclusion, to make the most of the advantages of intermittent fasting, it is essential to have a well-rounded and healthy lifestyle, which should include